Fernanda Teles

Electromyographic Parameters in Exercises with Elastic Resistance

Fernanda Teles

Electromyographic Parameters in Exercises with Elastic Resistance

Physiologically understand the importance of intensity control when exercising with elastic implements

ScienciaScripts

Cover image: www.ingimage.com

This book is a translation from the original published under ISBN 978-3-330-75794-3.

Publisher:
Sciencia Scripts
is a trademark of
Dodo Books Indian Ocean Ltd. and OmniScriptum S.R.L publishing group

120 High Road, East Finchley, London, N2 9ED, United Kingdom
Str. Armeneasca 28/1, office 1, Chisinau MD-2012, Republic of Moldova, Europe
Printed at: see last page
ISBN: 978-620-8-29262-1

CONTENTS

ACKNOWLEDGMENTS

"The world as we have created it is a process of our thinking. It cannot be changed without changing our thinking."

Albert Einstein

I am grateful for the opportunity to take a *stricto-sensu* specialization *course and* thus experience unique experiences in order to contribute to academic, social and professional knowledge.

To my parents, Vitória Elizabeth Sampaio Bastos and Sidnei Ribeiro Teles, who gave me the best possible education and supported me in my decisions; and to all my family members who have always supported me.

To my great advisors, professors and friends Marcelino Monteiro de Andrade and Jake Carvalho do Carmo, who have accompanied me throughout my academic career and allowed me to experience experiences whose teachings transcend those necessary to obtain this degree. I dedicate this entire work to them.

Gabriela Sartòrio Barbosa, Maria Clàudia Cardoso Pereira, Valdinar de Araùjo Rocha Jûnior, Filipe Barreto Tomé and David Fiorillo are friends who have always been there for me in times of achievement, collection and difficulty, and who have never refused any form of help when there have been unforeseen circumstances. With them I share the merits of completing the dissertation.

To all the staff and faculty of the Faculty of Physical Education, Faculty of Technology and Faculty of Gama of the University of Brasilia for taking care of my work environment over the years and adding value to my training and academic growth.

To the research volunteers for their availability, commitment and seriousness in carrying out the tests.

To all my friends who played an indirect role in my master's degree but who never failed to accompany, support and encourage me during these years.

SUMMARY

ELECTROMYOGRAPHIC parameters IN EXERCISES WITH RESISTANCE.

the aim of this study was to analyze the behavior of electromyographic parameters during elbow flexion performed with elastic resistance under objective or subjective load control. The electromyographic signal was recorded by a bipolar electrode in the biceps brachii muscle of 31 male subjects (29.03 ± 5.99 years, 81.81 ± 8.65 kg, 179.09 ± 5.05 cm) practicing resistance training. The subjects performed two maximal voluntary isometric contractions (MVC) with the elbow at 90 degrees and were allocated, in a counterbalanced manner, to either the *biofeedback* group (GBlo) or the subjective load control group (GTRD). All subjects performed three tasks with different resistances (pulley and elastic band). The tasks consisted of twelve unilateral repetitions of elbow flexion at 30% of CVIM. This intensity was used during the pulley exercise, with elastic resistance at the start of the movement and halfway through. The electromyographic variables were compared using mixed design factorial ANOVAs. For RMS, there was an interaction between groups and main effects between tasks. There were no significant differences between the GBlo tasks. Significant differences were found in the tasks that used elastic resistance compared to the pulley in the GTRD. For FPMd, there were no interactions or main effects. The Bland and Altman (1983) procedure confirmed agreement between all tasks for FPMd. Muscle activation was significantly modified when the exercise was performed without objective load control during elbow flexion with elastic resistance.

Keywords: surface electromyography, elastic resistance, load control.

CHAPTER 1 - INTRODUCTION

Resistance training (RT) is commonly used as a strategy for developing physical abilities and is practiced by many different populations. A variety of technologies are used to enable the practice of physical training according to the objective to be achieved (Fleck & Kraemer, 2006).

Exercises performed with free weights, pulleys or bodybuilding machines have constant resistance and can vary in speed of execution, number of repetitions, different muscle actions, among others. On the other hand, exercises practiced with variable resistance, such as elastic bands, have load variations during the execution of the movement (Fleck & Kraemer, 2006). Despite the variation in intensity, elastic bands have unique characteristics when compared to equipment with a constant load. They combine practicality, portability and low cost. However, the literature lacks studies comparing exercises performed with elastic implements and those with a constant load.

In addition to the few studies on elastic resistance, the difficulty in obtaining a methodological procedure capable of allowing a comparison between the types of resistance to be used and the physiological consequences for each intervention, makes the use of elastic implements restricted and aimed at joint rehabilitation or clinical programs, where the exercises are mostly performed at submaximal intensities (Andersen et al. 2010, Colado et al., 2011). According to Andersen et al. (2010) only a few studies have analyzed the physiological adaptations induced by elastic resistance exercises compared to other contraction modalities. In addition, previous studies have found that the use of elastic resistance at an appropriate intensity provides significant improvements in functional tests and causes changes in body composition with a reduction in abdominal perimetry and body fat percentage (Colado et al. 2008, 2009).

Despite the evidence in favor of elastic resistance, most of the materials available today do not objectively determine the intensity of the exercises.

Therefore, in order to control the level of intensity, subjective perception of exertion (PSE) scales are used. Colado and his colleagues (2012) validated such a scale for this purpose. In this study, the progressive increase in SPE during elastic resistance exercise was directly related to acute and increasing physiological adaptations in the muscular and cardiac systems. Even though we are aware of the benefits of using a PES scale, the lack of a method for quantitative and direct control of the intensity of elastic exercises does not allow us to establish clear dose-effect relationships, as has already been demonstrated by meta-analyses of TR with weights and pulleys (Steib et al., 2010; Peterson et al., 2010).

Surface electromyography (SEMG) has been a commonly used method for evaluating electromyographic activation related to the intensity of physical exercise. It is known that the use of SEMG can provide relevant information on the recruitment of motor units (Bonato et al., 1996) as well as the behavior of localized muscle fatigue (Gerleman et al. 1989). In addition, muscle electrical activity in RT can prove benefits, enhance results or correct any flaws in existing methods (Rocha Júnior, 2008). Some authors have used this tool, adding value to the discussion about neuromuscular behavior during exercises with different types of resistance (Cannon et al., 2007; Melchiorri et al., 2011; Calatayud et al. 2015).

In view of this problem, the creation of specific methods and protocols based on scientific evidence for reliable intensity control during elastic exercises is of fundamental importance.

1.1 Objective

The aim of this study was to analyze the behavior of electromyographic parameters during elbow flexion exercise performed with elastic resistance under objective or subjective load control. The aim was to verify whether the use of *biofeedback* and objective load control modify the pattern of muscle activation and fatigue during elbow flexion compared to the use of constant and variable resistance with subjective intensity control, i.e. based on the perception of effort.

1.2 Justification

The latest consensus on resistance training points to the effectiveness of machines and free weights for improving muscle function and body composition variables (ACSM 2009; Steib et al., 2010; Peterson et al., 2010). Elastic resistance studies have also shown beneficial outcomes for muscle function variables in different populations (Colado et al. 2008; Colado et al. 2010; Melchiorri et al., 2011, Martins, 2013; Calatayud et al. 2015).

However, there is a lack of studies in the literature that have compared exercises performed with constant resistance to exercises performed with variable resistance. This may be due to the difficulty in establishing a methodological consensus on load control using variable resistance. Normally, intervention protocols try to do this control qualitatively, i.e. using subjective perception of effort scales (Colado et al., 2012) or even using elastics with different resistance level information provided by the manufacturers themselves (Martins et al., 2013).

It is known that the recruitment behavior of motor units measured using surface electromyography can provide information on gains in muscle capacity in different populations (Cannon et al., 2007; Melchiorri et al., 2011). This tool can make a significant contribution to deepening our understanding of the need to control training load, because according to Gerleman et al. (1989) SEMG allows us to analyze the relationship between the electromyographic signal and force production.

In view of the above, the present study proposed a methodology in which the intensity of exercises practiced with elastic resistance was controlled by means of force transducers and *biofeedback*, in order to guarantee quantitative control of intensity during physical exercise. It is not to our knowledge that electromyographic parameters of amplitude and frequency have been studied during exercises using quantitative load control devices for elastic resistance. Correct manipulation of the intensity of elastic bands can transform these implements into an effective alternative for TR practitioners in various populations, reinforcing their portability and adding positive results for the development of physical capacities (Colado et al. 2008, 2010; Melchiorri et al., 2011; Calatayud et al. 2015).

CHAPTER 2 - LITERATURE REVIEW

2.1 Resistive Methods and Load Control

Resistance training can be defined as the practice of exercises that promote movements of body segments against a certain force usually exerted by some type of equipment (Fleck & Kraemer, 2006). The first scientific research appeared at the end of the 1940s when the authors Delmore and Watkins wrote about progressive intensity strength exercises in the rehabilitation of military personnel in the post-war period (Kraemer et al., 2002).

The application of resistance training requires the development of a training program which is considered a complex task as it requires knowledge and control of the variables that influence the practitioner's performance based on the objective to be achieved (Tan, 1999). In order to provide a general description of a session, acute variables are used, such as the choice of exercises, speed of execution, training overload, recovery interval, among others (Fleck & Kraemer, 2006).

Overload or load is definitely a key factor in any resistance training program because, in addition to determining a level of intensity, it is the main stimulus related to the changes observed in the measurements of strength and localized muscular endurance (Tan, 1999; Fleck & Kraemer, 2006). The variation in training intensity may be related to the different muscle actions. It is known that there are three types of muscle action: concentric, eccentric and isometric. The first consists of shortening the muscle, i.e. the contraction itself. The second consists of stretching the fibers in a controlled manner, referring to the return to the initial position of the exercise in question. Finally, the last consists of muscle activation without moving the joint that is being requested (Fleck & Kraemer, 2006; McArdle, 2008). Currently, there is also the isokinetic type of movement which, during concentric and eccentric action, has a constant speed (Azevedo, 2003; Bottaro et al., 2005). This type of speed control has proved to be a good option for muscle training and joint rehabilitation, as the performer must achieve the desired degree of strength and execute it throughout the movement at the required speed (Farina et al., 1999; Azevedo, 2003).

When analyzing dynamic contractions (concentric and eccentric actions) there are technologies that can directly influence the control of the intensity variable. Exercises performed on pulleys, free weights or machinery are characterized by exerting a constant load. Despite variations in the angles of mechanical advantage and disadvantage, the overload is the same from the beginning to the end of the movement. Elastic resistance exercises vary the load throughout the range of movement. This variation tries to accompany the increases and decreases in force during the range of movement by increasing or decreasing elastic deformation (Fleck & Kraemer, 2006; Martins et al., 2013). According to Sakanoue et al. (2007), the variation in resistance follows the force curve of the exercise where the active muscle is forced to contract increasingly throughout the range of movement.

Resistance training using constant loads is well described in the literature as it allows for intensity control. Studies that propose different exercise protocols are able to describe the increases in overload over the course of training weeks and explore the physiological and mechanical variables that influence gains in strength and/or muscle volume (Schoenfeld, 2010). Prestes et al. (2009) verified the effect of a 12-week training program with different periodization models on the strength levels and body composition of individuals practicing resistance training. Their study explains the importance of controlling intensity in resistance training with constant loads, where all the overloads used to carry out the experimental protocol were based on percentiles determined from the 1RM test, which determines the maximum overload to perform a given movement with the correct technique (Rocha Júnior, 2008). This made it possible to quantify the load to be used for each exercise and to monitor the intensity and volume on a weekly basis until the 12 sessions were completed.

The pulley, in particular, can have a variable radius configuration that "transforms" it into a resistive method with variable behavior, just like the elastic (figure 1). This variation in radius is intended to allow the torque generated by the exercise to increase (McMaster et al., 2009). Fleck and Kraemer (2004) described that for the elbow flexion exercise on pulleys of varying radius, the resistance offered in the middle of the range of movement is greater compared to the first portion and the last fourth movement.

Figura 1 - Variation of the radius of a pullover exercise machine (McMaster et al., 2009).

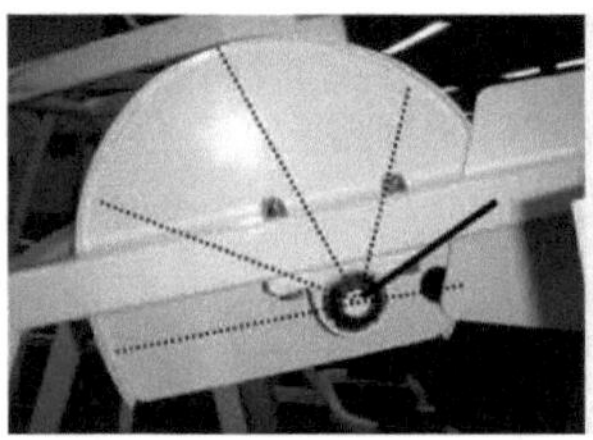
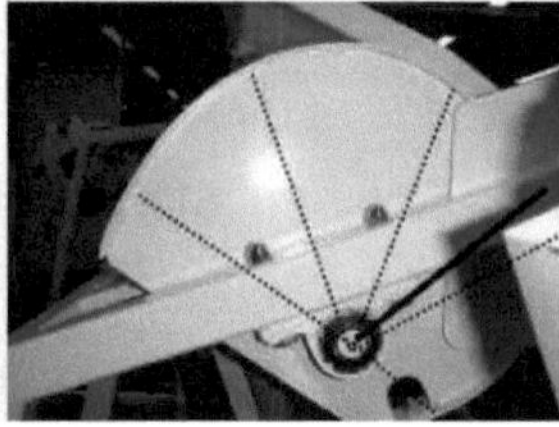
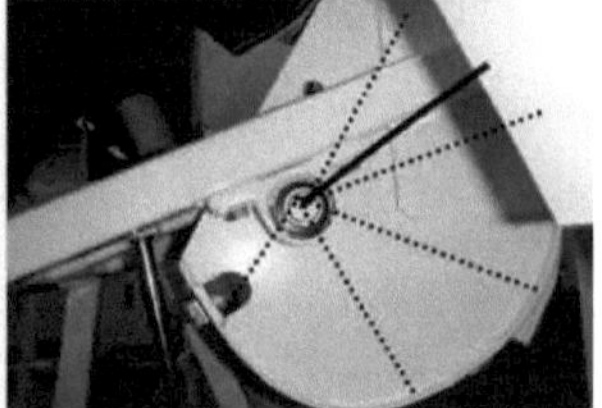

Highlighted, the radius of varying size in bold during the movement of the equipment

When associated with surface electromyography, many studies focus on variations in movement and the different machines, seeking to understand the mechanisms that help active muscles achieve certain levels of strength. As an example, the study by Schwanbeck et al. (2009) compared the muscle activation of the primary motors of the squat movement, as well as their stabilizers, using free weights and the Smith machine. As a result, he obtained a significant increase in the activation of the gastrocnemius, biceps femoris and vastus medialis muscles when using free weights compared to the machine. Using the same experimental design, Welsch et al. (2005) analyzed the electromyographic activity of the pectoralis major, clavicular and anterior deltoid muscles in the dumbbell bench press, barbell bench press and dumbbell crucifix. Differences in motor unit activation were not statistically significant for any of the three movements. However, there is a gap in studies comparing fixed resistance to variable resistance.

Considered an example of variable loading, elastic resistance has unique characteristics. Unlike the pulley, in which the force exerted offers less resistance at the end of the elbow flexion movement (Fleck & Kraemer, 2006), in elastic resistance, the intensity imposed, associated with the type of material and the levels of deformation achieved, becomes greater at the end of the range of movement (Simoneau et al., 2001). In a mechanical test carried out by Martins et al. (2014), it was found that commercial elastic bands in the form of tubes, commonly used for physical exercise, impose an increase in load directly proportional to the stretching of the material. This quantification of the load makes the use of the elastic implement more objective, making it easier to control the intensity. However, the elastic deformation behavior analyzed by the authors is very specific to a single type of elastic and brand. The reproducibility of these values for other types of implement was not carried out, thus maintaining the problem of the lack of quantitative load control for elastic bands.

In this context, load control for variable resistance becomes subjective and comparison with fixed resistance a challenge. According to Andersen et al. (2010) few studies have analyzed the physiological adaptations induced by elastic resistance exercises compared to other contraction modalities. In addition, previous studies have found that the use of elastic resistance at an appropriate intensity provides significant improvements in functional tests and causes changes in body composition with a reduction in abdominal perimetry and body fat percentage (Colado et al. 2008, 2009) in different populations. Jakobsen et al. (2014) compared the effectiveness of rehabilitating knee flexors in exercises performed with elastic resistance and weight training machines using surface electromyography. In their results, there was a similarity in muscle activation for both tasks, although the task with elastic overload showed higher values in perceived exertion when compared to the machine. The authors justified this result by the multiple degrees of freedom of the leg when performing the knee flexion movement. As for strength gains,

Calatayud et al. (2015) found similar gains through muscle activation levels and 1RM and 6RM tests for the bench press exercise performed with bars and washers compared to the arm flexion movement performed with elastic resistance.

However, the lack of consistent studies in the literature proposing methods and protocols capable of quantifying the intensity of exercises with variable load makes it difficult to standardize strength tests, as well as those already carried out with constant resistance. This hinders research into the physiological responses and biomechanical interactions arising from different overload methods (Azevedo, 2003; Martins, 2013).

In an attempt to control intensity more objectively, authors such as Fuller (1997), Hunter et al. (2001), Oliveira et al. (2009) and Melchiorri et al. (2011) propose the use of *biofeedback* to control acute RT variables. This technique comes from the phenomenon of "*feedback*", which is understood as a set of control mechanisms capable of adapting to routine or even physiological situations (Fuller, 1977). There are various ways of providing *feedback* to an exerciser. Moras et al. (2009) used a metronome to control the speed at which the bench press was performed at different intensities. These intensities were determined using the 1RM test for fixed resistance.

According to Rosa de Sà et al. (2012), *biofeedback* is an element of support that allows the practitioner, voluntarily or indirectly, to learn to control the body's physiological parameters. To do this, they need some means of providing the individual with biological information (muscle tension, skin temperature, brain activity, heart rate) and/or psychophysiological information (degree of stress, relaxation, arousal, anxiety) that they could not infer directly. This technique can range from a simple mirror to a sophisticated electronic device. The important thing is that the person is given immediate information about what is happening in their body at a given moment (Rosa de Sà et al., 2012).

The study by Melchiorri et al. (2011) describes the use of *biofeedback* to compare the force curve of different resistive methods. To indicate the intensity range in which the subject should perform the protocol, force transducers were connected to a *display* which provided the individual with visual *biofeedback* on the level of torque produced. Hunter et al. (2001) also used the visual *biofeedback* tool to provide information on the correct angulation of the elbow joint in one of the tasks performed in their experimental protocol.

In addition, perceived exertion (PSE) scales can also be used as *biofeedback* to assess the level of intensity during exercise (Robertson et al., 2003; McArdle, 2008). The study by Oliveira et al. (2009) compared the SEMG signal and heart rate with the results obtained using a subjective perception of effort scale in the elbow flexion movement in different positions (standing and sitting). The results found by these authors corroborate the use of this technique to assess levels of intensity. Martins (2013) used PSE to control the intensity of a muscle strength training program using elastic resistance in the elderly. This procedure exemplified the current context of using elastic resistance where load control during exercise is either non-existent or done using a subjective effort scale for elastic resistance (OMNI-RES) validated by Colado et al. 2012 and shown in figure 2.

Figura 2 - *OMNI resistance exercise scale of perceived exertion* for use with elastic bands (Colado et al. 2012).

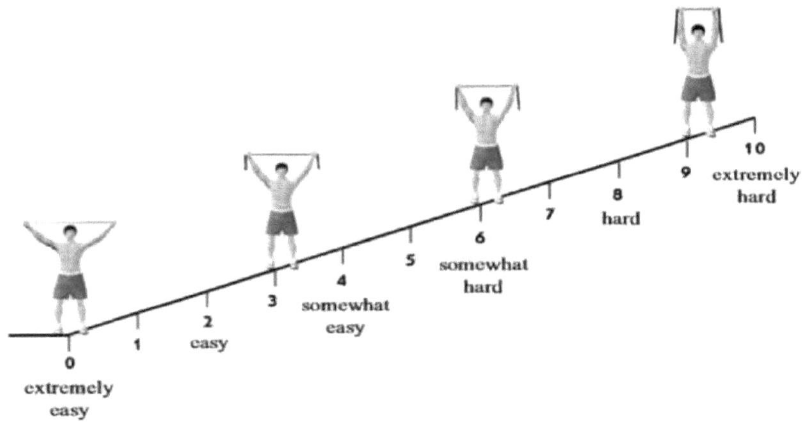

2.2 Electromyography

Electromyography (EMG) is a technique that consists of acquiring and processing the electrical signal produced in the muscles by stimulating motor units over time (Merletti and Parker, 2004). This technique enables inferences to be made about physiological properties such as muscle fatigue, as well as force production mechanisms (Anders et al., 2005). Electromyography also has two acquisition methods. One is invasive, where the electrodes are inserted directly into the muscles and are needle-shaped, or one is non-invasive, where the electrodes are positioned on the surface of the skin (De Luca, 1997). This technique can be affected by various factors such as muscular, anatomical and physiological properties, the control of the peripheral nervous system and the instrumentation used (Mezzarane et al., 2014).

In the case of surface electromyography (SEMG), the type of electrode, its shape and composition have a direct influence on signal capture and quality (De Luca, 1997; Merletti and Parker, 2004; Andrade, 2006; Rocha Júnior, 2008; Pereira, 2009). As a way of improving capture and minimizing noise, electrodes of a reasonable size are used to keep them in the belly of the muscle being analysed and which allow good contact with the skin (De Luca, 1997). Its composition is often chlorinated silver (Ag-AgCl) which offers low impedance to the skin and its operation is linked to a differential amplification system (Hermens et al., 2000). The bipolar electrode configuration has been commonly used and picks up different electromyographic signals via two contacts. During acquisition, an additional electrode is placed in a bone or tendon region close to the event being studied in order to use it as a signal reference common to all the electrodes. The differences in the signals obtained are then amplified, and this method is called simple differential amplification, as illustrated in figure 3. The common signal resulting from the differences between the signals obtained is then rejected (noise). The ability to reject the common signal is called the common mode rejection rate.

Figure 3 - Representation of the differential amplification of a bipolar electrode.

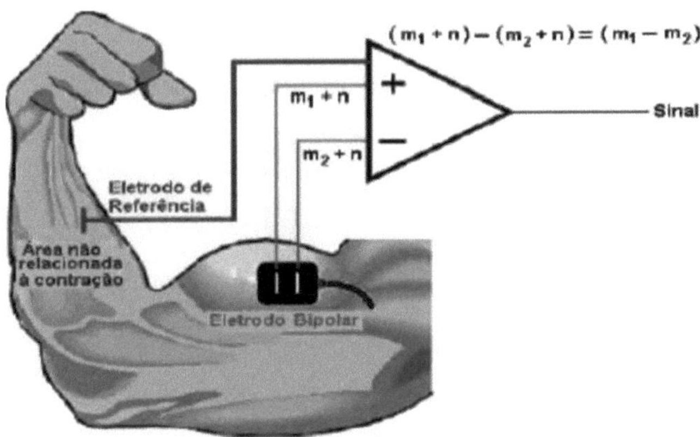

The electromyographic signals obtained are represented by "ml" and "m2", and the noise by "n" (modified - De Luca, 2002; Rocha Júnior, 2006).

Electrodes can also be classified as active or passive. Active electrodes are those that have an electronic circuit responsible for previously amplifying the signals captured before they reach the electromyograph (the instrument responsible for processing the electromyographic signal) (Marchetti et al., 2006). Prior amplification can be accompanied by signal filtering and the elimination of low and high frequency noise, i.e. noise related to movement artifacts or other types of noise. Passive electrodes are those that only capture the electromyographic signal, without any prior treatment until it reaches the electromyograph (Marchetti et al., 2006).

SENIAM (*Surface EMG for the Non-Invasive Assessment of Muscles)* has recommendations for the use and placement of surface electrodes as a way of standardizing their use and avoiding major harmful interferences with the location of motor points. It is known that the quality of the signal can be compromised by the capture of the cardiac electrical signal, *crosstalk* (electrical signal coming from muscles close to the muscle being studied), movement artifacts and the direction of the electrode in relation to the muscle fibers (De Luca, 1997). Figure 4 shows the changes in amplitude and frequency of the electromyographic signal captured by a bipolar electrode in different regions of the muscle.

Figure 4 - Changes in the SEMG amplitude signal and frequency spectrum as electrode placement varies (modified - De Luca, 1997).

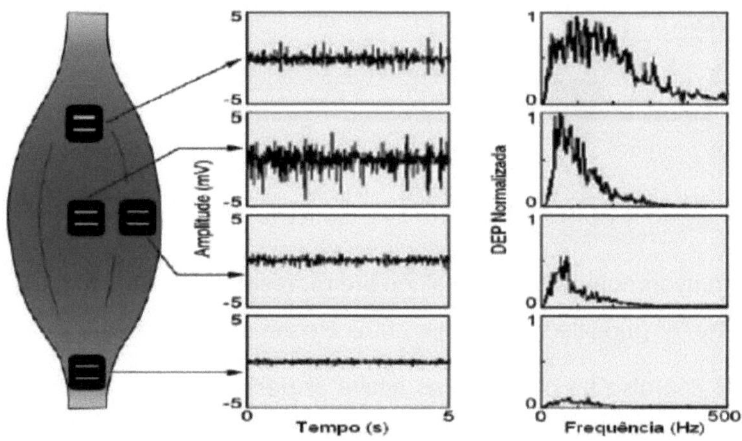

DEP is the power spectral density (modified - Andrade, 2006).

Although SENIAM's recommendations on the positioning of the electrode on the skin, prior procedures and the construction of the sensors are an attempt to minimize noise, it is known that noise-free acquisitions are impossible (Konrad, 2005). Researchers and clinicians should therefore be aware of the main sources of noise and seek solutions to minimize their occurrence.

In the case of dynamic contractions, it is known that the electrode moves over the skin in addition to muscle movement. These factors can generate movement artifacts with frequencies ranging from 0 to 20 Hz (Merletti and Parker, 2004). This type of noise can be minimized by correctly fixing the electrode to the skin and the cables connected to it. As a way of reducing skin impedance, abrasion and trichotomy procedures are adopted to improve signal capture in dynamic and isometric circumstances (Webster, 1984).

Electromagnetic fields are common sources of noise during the acquisition of surface electromyographic signals. In Brazil, this noise often comes from the

60Hz alternating current supplied by electricity operators and/or its harmonics. Normally, the amplitude of this signal is greater than that of the electromyographic signal (Andrade, 2006; Rocha Jûnior, 2008; Pereira, 2009). As a way of reducing its capture, Clancy et al. (2002) proposed different noise attenuation strategies. Suggestions such as using differential amplifiers and shielded accessories, in addition to keeping them intertwined, reduce their exposure to different ranges of electromagnetic fields. In addition, ensuring good grounding (environment and patient) and using *nobreaks* during acquisition corroborate the attempt to reduce noise capture.

The acquisition of surface electromyographic signals involves suitable *hardware* for differential amplification and common mode rejection. The analog signal emitted by the body must be converted into a digital signal using an analog-to-digital converter and recorded on the computer. This configuration requires adjustments such as sampling frequency, amplifiers, filters, analog-to-digital converter, among others (De Luca, 2002; Marchetti et al., 2006).

Converting an analog signal into a digital one requires parameters that enable correct reproduction so that appropriate inferences can be made. The sampling frequency consists of reading the signal at specific times associated with the sampling period (De Luca, 2003). If the signal is digitally reproduced at a low frequency, it may not contain all the relevant information (Erfanian et al. 1994, ; De Luca, 2003). The sampling frequency follows the theorem proposed by Nyquist which states that the reconstruction of the digital signal must use at least twice its highest frequency. In the case of electromyography, since the maximum frequency is 500Hz, the sampling frequency must be at least 1000Hz (De Luca, 2003). In the case of differential amplifiers and common mode rejection rates, a value of at least 100dB is recommended to guarantee and improve signal quality (Clancy et al., 2002; De Luca, 2003).

Filters are tools used to attenuate specific variations in frequency components, i.e. allowing the desired signal to be separated and restored (Carmo, 2003;

Rocha Jùnior, 2008). Separation is necessary when the signal has been contaminated by interference or noise. Restoration is used when the signal has been distorted (Marchetti et al., 2006). Applications of the electromyographic signal at frequencies above 500 Hz do not correspond to physiological factors, which in this case would be muscle contraction (Merletti and Parker, 2004). Therefore, bandpass filters with cut-off frequencies between 20 and 500 Hz are used for signal analysis (De Luca, 1997; Merletti and Parker, 2004). Filters can be analog or digital (De Luca, 2003).

The classic methods for analyzing the EMG signal can be summarized as time-domain and frequency-domain analysis. The information represented in the time domain describes when something occurs and the amplitude of its occurrence (Carmo, 2003; Pereira, 2009). This parameter can indicate the magnitude of muscle activity by the level of activation of recruited motor units and the firing rate of active motor units (Farina, 2004). The most common methods for interpreting the time-domain EMG signal are RMS and ARV (De Luca, 2002; Merletti and Parker, 2004). Amplification of the surface electromyographic signal is necessary given the amplitude variation of only 0 to 10 mV peak to peak (De Luca, 2002) and analysis of the raw signals can lead to erroneous inferences. Depending on the type of method chosen, prior procedures such as rectification and normalization of the signal are essential.

Complete rectification consists of eliminating the negative values of the signal by converting them into positive values, thus conserving the energy of the surface electromyographic signal (De Luca, 2006). This method is necessary because the amplitude of the raw signal varies between positive and negative values as they correspond to the phenomenon of polarization and depolarization of the muscle membrane and due to differential measurement. If the signal is not rectified, amplitude calculations can be underestimated and unrealistic.

Figure 5 - Raw and full-wave rectified electromyographic signal (Marchetti et

al., 2006)

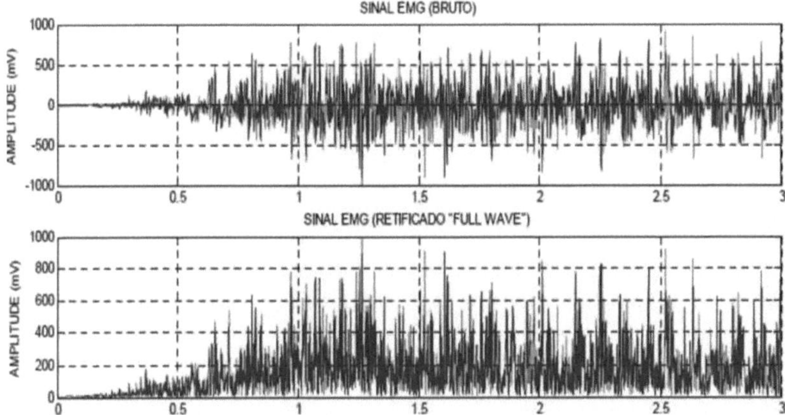

After rectifying the signal (figure 5), the normalization procedure consists of re-establishing the electromyographic signal's scale from a given reference. This procedure makes it possible to compare signals from different subjects and/or groups (Marchetti et al., 2006) and can be done in three different ways. The first of these uses the maximum isometric voluntary contraction (MIVC) as a reference, where the signal from this contraction is defined as 100% of muscle electrical activity and the other values on the scale are converted into percentages relative to this maximum (De Luca, 1997). Other forms of normalization are based on the average or maximum value of the signal itself.

After rectifying and normalizing the signal, respectively, the muscle activation level is calculated using the *Root Mean Square* (RMS) method or the *Average Rectified Value* (ARV). To calculate the RMS value, all the samples of the SEMG signal are summed to the second power. This sum is divided by the total number of samples and the square root of the obtained quotient is extracted (De Luca, 1997). ARV consists of the sum of the rectified signal over a time interval, divided by the size of the interval (Merletti et al., 1999). Equations 1 and 2 show how to find these SEMG signal amplitude estimates for the m-th signal window.

$$\mathrm{RMS}(m) = \sqrt{\frac{1}{N}\sum_{n=0}^{mN-1}|f(n)^2|} \tag{1}$$

$$\mathrm{ARV}(m) = \frac{1}{N}\sum_{n=0}^{mN-1}|f(n)| \tag{2}$$

Although these mathematical tools are similar and allow inferences to be made about the level of muscle activation (Merletti et al., 1999, De Luca 2002, Konrad, 2005) and/or associations between signal amplitude and physical valences, the RMS value is well-established in the literature and consistently demonstrates linearity for both dynamic and isometric contractions in relation to the amplitude of the electromyographic signal (Moritani et al., 1987; De Luca, 1997; Alkner et al., Masuda et al., 2001; Bilodeau et al., 2003).

In the frequency domain, the SEMG is represented in a frequency spectrum, where the signal content is represented as a histogram and normally using the Fast Fourier Transform (Moritani et al., 1987; Christensen et al., 1995; Andrade, 2006). Physiologically, there are some parameters that can influence the representation of this signal in the frequency domain, such as the firing rate of the motor units, the relative firing time of the action potentials by different motor units and the shape of the action potentials (Carmo, 2003; Pereira, 2009; Rocha Jùnior, 2008; Soares, 2013). These changes can be inferred in the presence of localized muscle fatigue, which originates in a defined muscle region that has been subjected to intense physical activity for a certain period of time (Chaffin, 1973).

Identifying patterns associated with muscle fatigue during isometric and dynamic contractions using SEMG is an important area of research into the motor system. In this sense, numerous techniques and protocols have been established in an attempt to understand or even standardize a behavior or adaptation to training (Carmo, 2003). Gelerman et al. (1996) and Lindstrom et al. (1970) showed that the presence of localized muscle fatigue gives a spectral signature to the SEMG signal with the presence of a decline in amplitude of the action potentials and an increase in their duration, shifting the frequency spectrum graph to the left.

The most commonly used frequency estimators for the SEMG signal are the mean power frequency (MPF) and median power frequency (MPFd). The FPMd estimator is usually used because it is less sensitive to noise and more sensitive to fatigue, which is desired in many studies (Soares, 2013). The FPMd estimator is calculated for the *m-th* window of the SEMG signal by finding the smallest value of km such that

$$\sum_{k=0}^{Km} |Fm(k)|^2 \geq \frac{1}{2} \sum_{k=0}^{N/2} |Fm(k)|^2 \tag{3}$$

and then calculating FPMd(m) = $fs(Km/N)$, where fs *is the* sampling frequency (in Hz), $Fm(k)$ is the discrete Fourier transform of the *m-th* signal window and N is the number of samples in the window (Soares, 2013).

Christensen et al. (1995) also stated that the RMS and FPMd values are increasing and decreasing, respectively, for isometric contractions. Physiologically, this spectral signature can be explained by the additional recruitment of motor units and/or increased synchronization and decreased firing rate, changes in synchronization and decreased conduction velocity (Andrade, 2006). In the case of dynamic contractions, Merletti and Parker (2004) and Bonato et al. (1996) associate the difficulty in not finding spectral patterns for muscle fatigue parameters with the non-stationarity of the myoelectric signal due to changes in muscle length and movement artifacts.

CHAPTER 3 - MATERIALS AND METHODS

3.1 Sample

The convenience sample consisted of 31 healthy males (age: 29.03 ± 5.99 years, mass: 81.81 ± 8.65 kg, height: 179.09 ± 5.05 cm). The volunteers had at least six months' experience in resistance training and consented to take part in the study after signing a consent form which explained all the methodological procedures, risks and benefits, as well as warning them that they could withdraw or abandon their participation of their own free will (ICF - Appendix I). Exclusion criteria were the presence of chronic diseases or injuries related to the musculoskeletal system or any other pathology that could hinder participation in the study. The project was approved by the Research Ethics Committee (CEP) of the Faculty of Health Sciences (CAAE: 16303013.0.0000.0030).

3.2 Introduction to Experimental Protocols

Resistance training has several variables that interfere acutely and/or chronically in the development of physical abilities. The exercise load is an example of a variable that the performer must fulfill during the execution of a task (Fleck & Kraemer, 2006). In this way, controlling the load allows the practitioner not only to monitor the evolution of their training, but also to take immediate action on the movement pattern and execution technique to fulfill the task in terms of intensity and training volume (Tan, 1999).

When training with free weights, pulleys or machines, the load is constant but the torque is variable. The changes in intensity vary according to the levers of the body members, i.e. although the load is the same from the beginning to the end of the movement, there are angular variations which generate greater or lesser mechanical disadvantages (Hall, 2000). However, in training using elastic resistance, this principle is modified by varying the load. In the case of elastic, as the deformation caused is greater, there is a progressive increase in the load (Martins et al., 2014).

In order to compare and standardize the intensity used in exercises with a fixed and variable load (elastic), the protocols applied in the study sought to reproduce two similar tasks in terms of overload. The task performed on the pulley represents the exercise being performed with a constant load and was used as a standard for comparison with the tasks performed with elastic resistance. Thus, all individuals, whether from GBIO or GTRD, performed it. The pulley task was also used to familiarize them with the test load.

The elastic resistance tasks were performed in two different ways. In the *biofeedback* group (GBIO), the tasks were performed using audio and visual *biofeedback*, ensuring that the performer was within the variable load range requested. In the traditional group (GTRD), the tasks with elastic resistance depended on the performer's own subjective perception of effort, which is the method most commonly used today.

3.3 Description of Experimental Protocols

In order to answer questions about the pattern of muscle recruitment and fatigue during exercises performed with different types of resistance and also to enable quantitative load control for elastic implements by means of *biofeedback*, this study devised a methodology which makes it possible to make inferences about electromyographic variables and statistically answer the proposed objective in relation to quantification and load control for elastic resistance.

All the protocols were carried out at the Biological Signal Processing and Motor Control Laboratory of the Faculty of Physical Education of the University of Brasilia (FEF/UnB). The protocols consisted of performing twelve (12) repetitions of the elbow flexion movement at 30% of CVIM on a low pulley (Gervasport *fitness equipment®)* or with elastic implements (Elastos®).

The volunteers were allocated to two groups in a counterbalanced manner: a group with objective load control and *biofeedback* (GBIO, n=16) or a group with subjective load control (GTRD, n=15).

All the volunteers performed three different tasks. The first, used as a standard for comparison, was performed on the pulley with 30% of the CVIM load. This task had to be the first in order to familiarize the subject with the load that would also be used in the elastic resistance task. The other tasks with elastic resistance were performed with 30% of the CVIM load at the start of the movement (elbow angle at maximum extension) called BIOi, where the "i" indicates start, and the other task with 30% of the CVIM load in the middle of the movement (elbow angle at approximately 90 degrees) called BIOm, where the "m" indicates middle. The order of the elastic resistance tasks was counterbalanced and a 10-minute interval was given between them (Melchiorri et al., 2001).

The variable resistance control device with *biofeedback* used in this study for the GBIO group works according to a range, in kilograms, previously programmed to be reached. In the case of the experimental protocol, as soon as 30% of the CVIM was reached, the device emitted visual *feedback* via a green LED and audible *feedback* warning that the subject had reached the proposed load. If the subject did not reach the programmed limit, the LED changed color to red and a continuous beep sounded simultaneously.

The GTRD participants performed the same three tasks as the GBIO, starting with the pulley (figure 6). However, in order to control intensity during the elastic tasks, the subjects positioned themselves according to their perception of effort in order to reach the proposed load for the tasks performed. For the traditional group, TRDi was the task in which the volunteers believed they had reached 30% of the CVIM at the start of the movement and TRDm when this same load was reached during the middle of the movement. The experimental protocol is summarized in figure 7.

Figura 6 - Pulley (TRDp) and elastic resistance (TRDi) tasks for the Traditional

Group (GTRD), respectively.

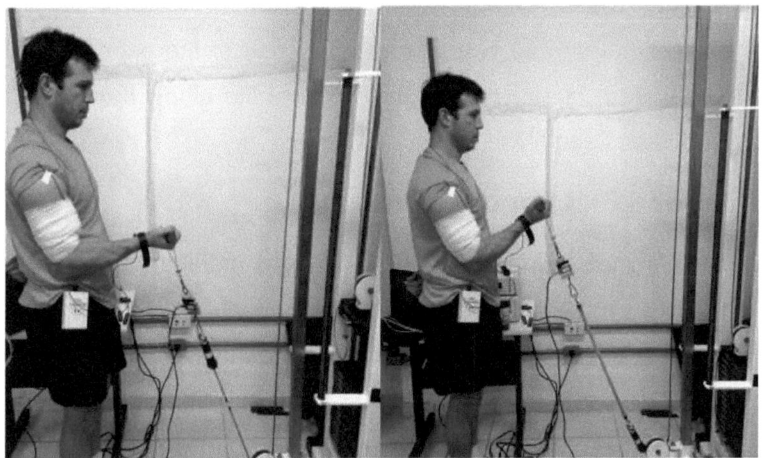

Figura 7 - Diagram of the research experimental protocols.

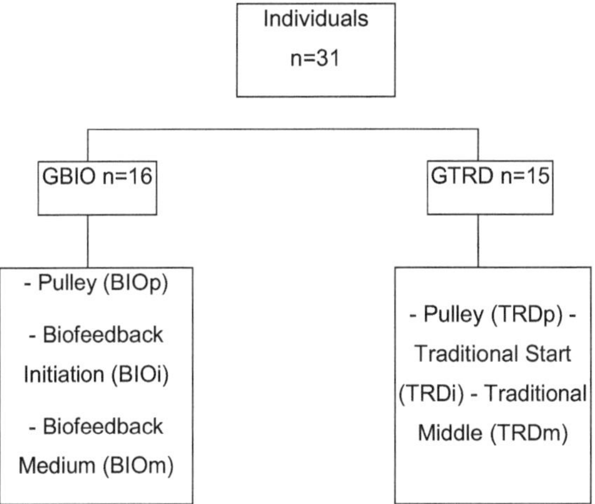

The elbow flexion repetitions were performed with the dominant arm at a pace pre-established by a metronome of two seconds for the concentric phase and two seconds for the eccentric phase (2020) (Melchiorri et al., 2001).

3.4 Procedures

After arriving at the laboratory, all the procedures were explained to the volunteers and they signed an informed consent form before the samples were taken. Anthropometric measurements were then taken to characterize the sample. After the volunteers had been allocated to one of the experimental groups, they underwent a test to assess the CVIM of the elbow flexors and determine the load to be used for the tasks.

3.4.1 Load Cell and Electrogoniometer

To acquire the force signals, a load cell (AEPH do Brasil Indùstria e Comércio Ltda., model TS, 50kg ±10%) was used during the CVIM during the tasks with fixed resistance for both groups and elastic resistance only for the GTRD group. For the GBIO group's elastic resistance tasks, a load cell (Interface, model SSM-ARS, 20kgf ±10%) specific to the *hardware* used in this study was used.

Both load cells were calibrated by applying known forces on the vertical axis to the cells. From the electrical voltages generated by the applied forces, the signals were processed in MatLab 6.5 (Mathworks; Natick, MA, USA) and a calibration curve was plotted for each cell.

The electrogoniometer made in-house at the Biological Signal Processing Laboratory - UnB was calibrated by coupling it to an analog goniometer at angles of 20, 30, 50, 60, 70, 90, 110, 130, 150, 170 and 180 degrees. These signals were processed in MatLab 6.5 (Mathworks; Natick, MA, USA) using specific routines developed for the instrument.

3.4.2 Anthropometric Assessment

Anthropometric measurements of body mass and height, defined as follows, were used to characterize the sample: - Body mass: is the set of organic and inorganic matter that makes up the different types of tissues and body elements (Guedes and Guedes, 2006). A digital electronic scale (Lider Balanças®, model *P180M)* with a resolution of 100 grams was used to measure mass.

- Height: refers to the distance between two planes tangential to the vertex and the soles of the feet when the individual is standing, in maximum inspiratory apnea (Guedes and Guedes, 2006). A stadiometer (Sanny®) with a resolution of one millimeter was used.

3.4.3 Maximum Isometric Voluntary Contraction

The maximum voluntary isometric contraction (MVIC) of the elbow flexors was acquired with the volunteer sitting on a chair with a specific backrest for the arm and with the elbow flexed to 90 degrees (figure 7). An analog goniometer (TTK, model 1216) was used to measure this angle.

The load cell (AEPH do Brasil Indùstria e Comércio Ltda., model TS, 50kg ±10%) was attached to the right foot of the chair and had a handle attached to its end by an inextensible iron chain, as shown in figure 7. This strap was adjusted so that the subject could maintain 90 degrees of elbow flexion and simultaneously print their maximum isometric force for five seconds in two attempts with a two-minute recovery interval (Melchiorri et al., 2011). The highest force value was used and its signal processed by a specific algorithm developed in MatLab 6.5 (Mathworks; Natick, MA, USA) in order to estimate the 30% CVIM value.

Figure 8 - Acquisition of maximum isometric voluntary contraction (MIVC).

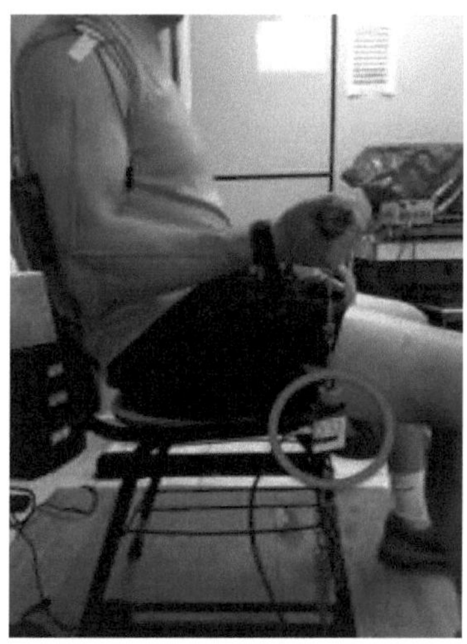

The load cell and elbow angle are highlighted.

3.4.4 *Biofeedback* device

The equipment for load control in exercises with elastic resistance and *biofeedback* (figure 8) controls, monitors and determines the load ranges, shown on a display, that the subject should perform during the exercise protocol. This equipment consists of a dynamometer with an on-board electronic system coupled to a load cell and has a patent registered with the National Institute of Industrial Property (INPI) under registration number BR 1020140072322 and is owned by the University of Brasilia Foundation (FUB).

This device was created to provide objective control in exercises with elastic implements and allows space-time variables to be converted by the system, optimizing intensity control (Andrade, 2014).

The electronic system is made up of a conditioning and acquisition center, which digitally processes the signal from a force sensor attached to the equipment, a processing center and the audio and visual *biofeedback* that guarantees the integration of the information from this sensor.

Its operation depends on three stages:

1. Physical exercise practiced by the user and the amount of force applied to the elastic implement;

2. Data related to this amount of force is acquired and processed according to the variables selected by the user on the device;

3. Provide *feedback* to the user on the execution of their movement and programmed intensity.

To set the value for 30% of CVIM on the *biofeedback* device, the evaluator rounded up or down the whole value when necessary, since the device had a unit scale in kilograms. For example, if the 30% value of the test subject's CVIM was 7.3 kg, the device was programmed for 7 kg during the elastic resistance tasks. If the value was greater than or equal to 7.5kg, the device was programmed to start the intensity range at 8kg.

Figure 9 - Load control equipment for elastic resistance with *biofeedback* adjusted for the tasks performed with the elastic implement in the GBIO.

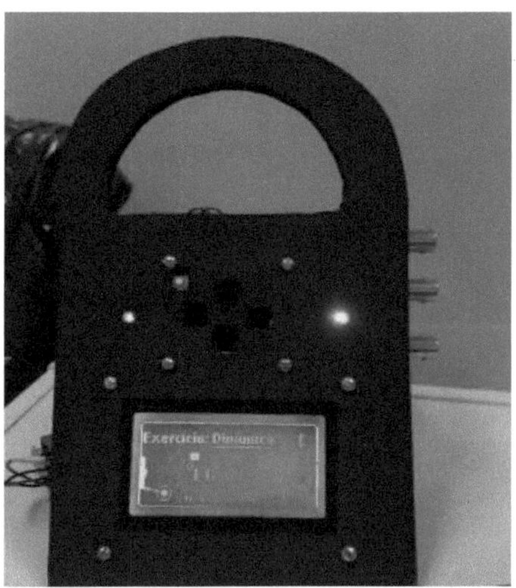

3.4.5 Elastic Resistance Equipment

The Elastos® brand has a kit with seven elastics of different colors and thicknesses that indicate their intensity (figure 9). The greater the thickness, the greater the force imposed to achieve the same elastic deformation. They are in order of intensity: yellow, red, green, blue, black, grape, gold.

Due to the characteristics of elastic resistance, only a range is determined where the target load is reached and not throughout the entire movement as occurs with fixed resistance (Melchiorri et al., 2011).

Figure 10 - Kit of Elastos® brand elastics and accessories used in this study.

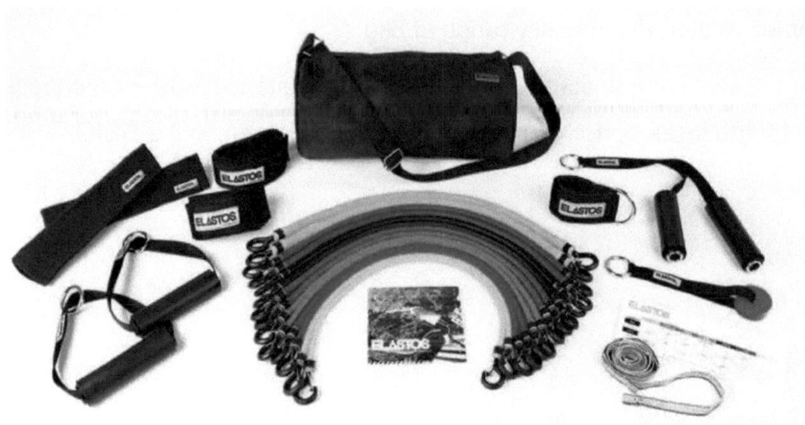

The choice of elastic strength based on the 30% CVIM load was determined using a load table developed by Martins et al. (2013) for Elastos®. This table provides a quantified value in kilograms of force (kgf) for each color of elastic based on a stretch of 50%, 100%, 150% and 200% of its initial size. We chose to use a stretch of 100% due to the possible sensation of discomfort when exercising with a large elastic deformation, giving the volunteer the impression that the elastics could burst.

3.4.6 Acquisition of Electromyography Signals

A bipolar electrode was attached to the long head of the biceps brachii muscle at 1/3 of the distance between the medial acromion and the cubital fossa, according to the SENIAM recommendations (Hermens et al., 2000).

A Delsys® electromyograph (model Bagnoli-2, Boston, USA) was used to acquire the electromyographic signals. Active electrodes were used with 10 V/V pre-amplification and a 20Hz to 450Hz band-pass filter. The total signal gain was 1000 V/V, with 10 V/V from the electrodes and 100 V/V from the electromyograph. The distance between electrodes was 1cm with chlorinated silver contacts (Ag-AgCl).

The signal obtained by the electromyograph was transferred to the computer using a 12-bit digital analog card (National Instruments, model PCI 6024E,

Austin, USA). The signals were acquired using the LabView computer tool and processed using MatLab version 6.5 (Mathworks; Natick, MA, USA).

The amplitude of the movement was controlled by an electrogoniometer previously specified in section 3.4.1. The signal obtained was used to cut out the concentric phase of the movement, considering 180° for complete elbow extension.

3.4.7 Signal Processing

The SEMG signal was initially filtered using a fourth-order *Butterworth* filter with a passband of 20 Hz to 500 Hz and phase delay correction (De Luca, 1997). A low-pass filter with the same characteristics and a cut-off frequency of 15 Hz was used to filter the force signal (Aagaard et al., 2000).

The electrogoniometer signal was used to cut out the heart sounds from the electromyographic signal in each repetition. The waves were delimited considering the entire concentric phase of the movement (figure 10). The first and last contractions were discarded from the analysis in order to minimize possible cadence maintenance problems that are common in the

at the beginning and end of the exercise series (Rocha Júnior, 2008).

Figure 11 - Representation of the clipping of the electromyographic signal based on information from the electrogoniometer.

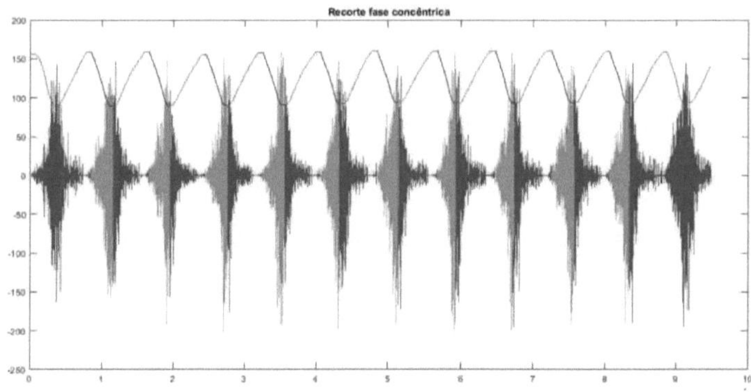

Highlighted (green), the concentric phase analyzed.

After normalizing the EMG signal by the maximum force signal obtained during the CVIM, the RMS and FPMd were calculated for each wave of each repetition according to equations 1 and 3, respectively. From the FPMd for each repetition, linear regressions were plotted to indicate the fatigue behavior triggered by the exercise. The slopes of the regression lines (angular coefficients) were normalized by their initial values (linear coefficients) to facilitate comparison between volunteers and experimental situations. All signal processing was done using specific routines developed in MatLab 6.5 software (Mathworks; Natick, MA, USA).

3.5 Statistical analysis

Elements of exploratory statistics were used to identify *outliers* and possible typing errors. Mean and standard deviation measurements were used to characterize the sample. A paired t-test was used to compare anthropometric data (mass, height and BMI) and age.

The Shapiro-Wilk test was used to verify the normality of the data, and Levene's test was used for equality of variances (Field, 2009). Once normality had been confirmed, intra-group comparisons of electromyographic variables (RMS and FPMd) were made using a 2x3 mixed factorial ANOVA [groups (GBIO, GTRD) x tasks (Pulley, Stretch-Start, Stretch-Middle)] (Field, 2009).

The intra-group comparisons are described in Table 1.

Table 1 - Summary of intra-group statistical comparisons.

GBIO	GTRD
BIOi x **BIOp**	TRDi x **TRDp**
BIOm x **BIOp**	TRDm x **TRDp**
BIOi x **BIOm**	TRDi x **TRDm**

BIOi = *biofeedback* task start; BIOm = *biofeedback* task middle; BIOp = *biofeedback* group pulley task; TRDi = traditional task start; TRDm = traditional task middle and TRDp = traditional group pulley task.

Due to the confirmation of non-significance in Levene's test, Turkey's post-hoc test was used to locate possible significant differences (Field, 2009).

Graphical analyses for the FPMd variable were carried out using the Bland-Altman (1986) graphical method. This tool makes it possible to compare two different methods and/or determine whether one of them can replace the one already established as the gold standard (Myles et al., 2007). Thus, the comparisons made used the pulley as the standard method, as it has a fixed and known load control.

All statistical analysis was carried out using SPSS software version 20.0.

CHAPTER 4 - RESULTS

The data for characterizing the sample is shown in Table 2. No significant differences were found for these values between the groups studied.

Table 2 - Description of the participants who made up the sample.

Variable	Mean ± standard deviation
n	31
Age (years)	29,03 ± 5,99
Mass (kg)	81,81 ± 8,65
Height (cm)	179,09 ± 5,05
body mass index (Kg/m)^2	25,52 ± 2,55

For the electromyography data, there was no loss of signal. We observed that the robustness of the equipment for acquiring electromyographic signals, together with all the previous procedures involving skin preparation, sample selection and minimizing environmental interference, were taken into account throughout the experimental protocol.

For the RMS values, there was an interaction between the groups (p=0.000) and a main effect for the tasks only within the traditional group (GTRD).

In the *biofeedback* group (GBIO), no significant differences were found in the RMS between the tasks with the BIOi (p=0.426) and BIOm (p=1.000) elastics compared to the pulley (BIOp). When compared to each other, the beginning (BIOi) and middle (BIOm) elastic tasks also showed no significant difference (p=0.157). It was observed that in the task with elastic and *biofeedback* for a load equivalent to 30% of the CVIM at the start of the movement, the RMS value was 9.85% higher than that found on the pulley. On the other hand, for the task with elastic and *biofeedback* for the load in the middle of the movement, there was a 0.4% decrease in the RMS value compared to the exercise performed on the pulley.

In the traditional group (GTRD), significant differences were found in the RMS between the TRDi (p=0.001) and TRDm (p=0.000) elastic tasks compared to the pulley (TRDp). When compared to each other, the beginning (TRDi) and middle (TRDm) elastic tasks also showed no significant difference (p=0.254) as in the GBIO. For the task with an elastic band and subjective control of the load equivalent to 30% of the CVIM at the start of the movement, the RMS value was 25.36% lower than that found on the pulley. Also in the task with an elastic band and subjective load control for the middle of the movement, it was possible to observe a 34.01% decrease in the RMS value compared to the exercise performed on the pulley.

There was no interaction (p=0.440) or main effect for the groups (p=0.767) and tasks (p=1.000). The mean values and standard deviation of the slopes of the regression lines were, for the GBIO pulley, elastic start and elastic middle tasks: -0.060 ± 0.05; -0.085 ± 0.15; -0.047 ± 0.03, respectively. For the GTRD, the average values of these inclinations were: -0.055 ± 0.04; 0.029 ± 0.52; -0.054 ± 0.05 for pulley, start elastic and middle elastic, respectively.

All the comparisons obtained by the graphical method proposed by Bland and Altman (1986) for the angular coefficients of the regression lines of the FPMd variable showed 96.7% of their values within the limit of agreement between the tasks performed with the elastic compared to the pulley. This statistical approach confirmed the good agreement between the proposed methods in terms of muscle fatigue. The comparisons are shown in figures 11 to 14.

Figura 12 - *Bland and Altman* graph with the PMFd values of the pulley and elastic start tasks for the GBIO group.

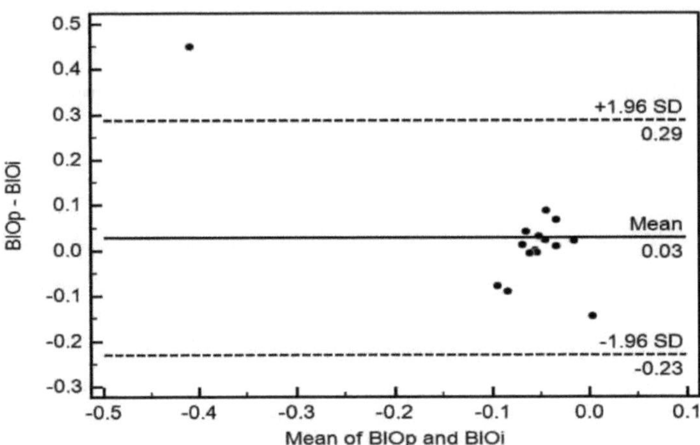

Figura 13 - *Bland and Altman* graph with the FPMd values of the pulley and middle elastic tasks for the GBIO group.

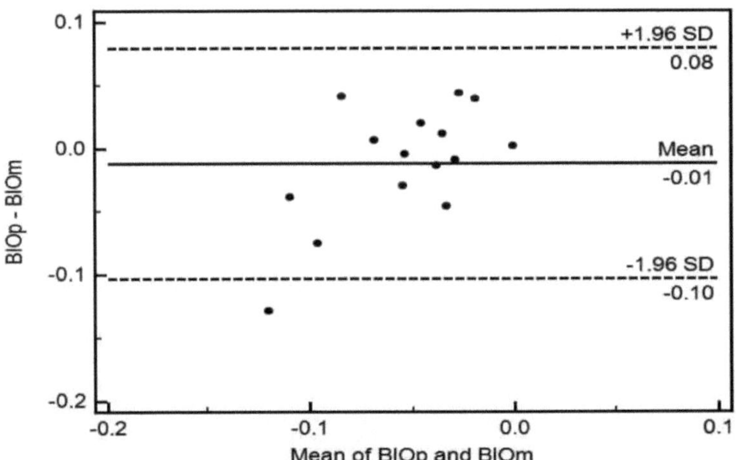

Figura 14 - *Bland and Altman* graph with the PMF values of the pulley and elastic start tasks for the GTRD group.

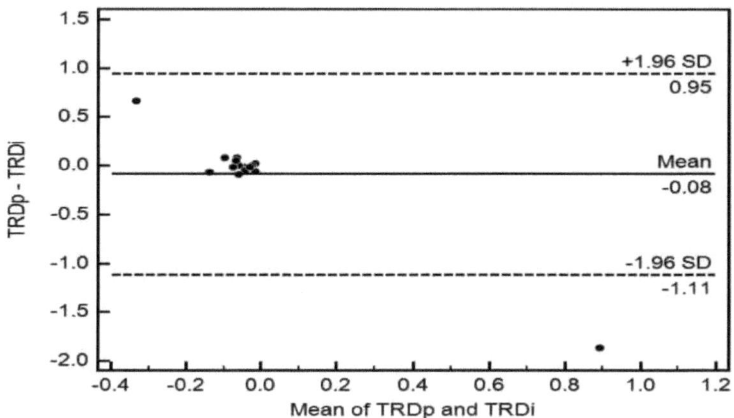

Figura 15 - *Bland and Altman* graph with the values of the FPMd of the pulley and middle elastic tasks of the GTRD group.

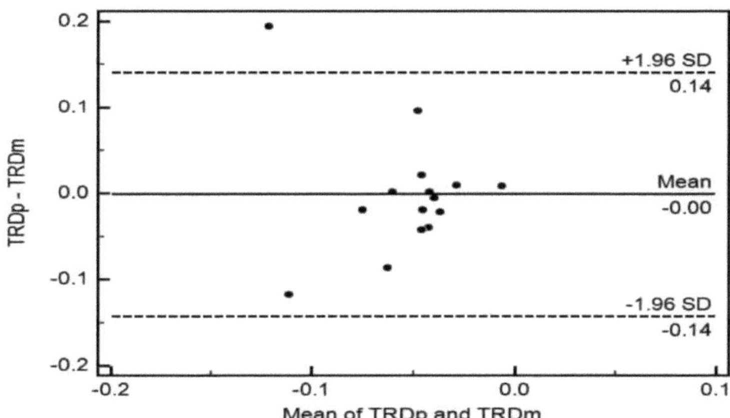

CHAPTER 5 - DISCUSSION

The aim of this study was to analyze the behavior of electromyographic parameters during elbow flexion exercise performed with elastic resistance under objective or subjective load control. It was expected that the use of objective load control for elastic implements with *biofeedback* would modify the pattern of muscle activation when compared to constant resistance and intensity control based on subjective perception of effort.

Another expected characteristic was that the tasks with elastic implements controlled by the subjective perception of effort would have their load underestimated even though the sample was characterized by active resistance trainers. As for muscle fatigue, it was expected that in no task in either group would this parameter interfere in such a way as to stop the activity or fail to sustain the imposed pace. However, it was speculated that the tasks with elastic implements might be more indicative of fatigue, especially in the group with the *biofeedback* load control device.

The analysis of the variation in electromyographic parameters using normalized slope lines is a procedure commonly described in the literature (Farina et al. 2004c; Andrade, 2006; Rocha Júnior, 2008). The signal recording and data processing used in this study are very similar to those used by Sundstrup et al. (2012). Although in their study they used upper limb muscles other than the biceps brachii, the recruitment parameters (amplitude) and frequency of the electromyographic signal during exercises performed with elastic implements at different intensities are similar to some of the results obtained in this dissertation.

The RMS value, i.e. the time-domain analysis variable of the electromyographic signal, is related to the recruitment of motor units during the exercise. The protocol carried out in the study sought to compare this variable with different types of resistance in a task with a fixed number of repetitions (12, in this case) and a low intensity (30% of CVIM, in this case). Although not exhaustive, the RMS variable in the GBIO group showed higher values (9.85%) in the beginning task (BIOi) when compared to the pulley task (BIOp). According to Bilodeau et al. (2003), the possible cause of this additional demand on motor units was compensation for the loss of contractile potential in the fibers that were initially demanded. In addition, the variable resistance increases in intensity during the concentric phase where the elastic deformation caused is directly proportional to the increase in load (Martins et al., 2014). Thus, the use of the load control device in the starting task (BIOi) ensures that the exercise starts at 30% of the CVIM but the concentric phase ends at a higher value than the one started. In the case of the pulley (BIOp), there is no variation in the load but only in the torque at different movement amplitudes (Leedham et al., 1995).

Despite the different and unique characteristics of the variable resistance, the load control and *biofeedback* device used in the GBIO ensured load control in the BIOi and BIOm tasks, as statistically there were no significant differences in the pattern of muscle recruitment when compared to the BIOp pulley task. The results of this study showed that the load, even though variable for the elastic implements, was sufficiently the same for all three tasks, reaching the level of intensity proposed by the protocol (30% of CVIM). In contrast, when we analyzed the RMS values of the traditional group (GTRD), which had subjective load control, the significant differences obtained in the comparisons of the tasks using elastic implements (TRDi and TRDm) in relation to the pulley (TRDp) show that the requested load was not only not reached, but was significantly underestimated. As a result, it was observed that the electronic system of the load control device with *biofeedback* was able to modify the movement pattern of the volunteers during the exercise practiced with elastic resistance and made it possible for spatio-temporal variables to be converted by the system, optimizing intensity control. The absence of load control for variable resistance is already reported as a problem in the study by Manning et al. (1989). The results obtained by these authors showed that the use of elastic resistance was insufficient to generate significant changes in isometric knee extension muscle strength compared to fixed resistance in young adults. In their arguments, they suggest that the absence of significantly positive results for the use of elastic resistance may, among other factors, be associated with the subjective load control used during the interventions. With the same argument regarding the lack of intensity control for elastic resistance, Martins (2013) justifies the lack of significance in his results following an eight-week physical training program using variable resistance in the elderly. Thus, the load control and *biofeedback* device is capable of modifying the movement pattern during elastic resistance exercise and enables spatio-temporal variables to be converted by the system, optimizing intensity control (Andrade, 2014).

Previous studies comparing elastic resistance and fixed resistance and/or investigating the behavior of elastic resistance at different intensities have sought to adapt training variables to these different resistances and evaluate physiological and functional aspects that result in gains in strength and resistance to muscle fatigue (Azevedo, 2003; Anderson et al., 2008; Andersen et al, 2010; Melchiorri et al., 2011; Colado et al., 2011; Sundstrup et al., 2012; Calatayude et al., 2015). Sundstrup et al. (2012) investigated recruitment strategies for the medial deltoid, upper trapezius, splenius and infraspinatus muscles using SEMG during the lateral shoulder raise exercise performed with maximum and submaximal loads using an elastic implement. The results showed that the greatest muscle activation (peak RMS value) occurred when the volunteers performed the submaximal load protocol compared to the maximum load protocol. Furthermore, this "maximum activation" occurred around 3-5 repetitions before the movement's concentric failure, i.e. if the individual performed 15 repetitions, their highest RMS value occurred around the tenth repetition. As in the study by Sundstrup et al. (2012), the load used in this study was 30% of the CVIM, i.e. a load considered submaximal. This common result reinforces the usability of the elastic implement in promoting higher levels of muscle activation in submaximal exercises. In addition, the results for muscle activation found in the present study during the activity performed with elastic resistance and objective load control (BIOi) showed similarly higher values compared to the pulley (9.85%).

In the case of the lower limbs, Jakobsen et al. (2013) analyzed the electromyographic signal of the muscles considered to be the primary motors and stabilizers of the forward exercise using dumbbells and elastic bands. Intensities of 33%, 66% and 100% were used in relation to the load of ten maximum repetitions (10RM). It was concluded that the greatest muscle recruitment of the hip and knee muscles occurred with the use of elastic resistance at medium intensity (66% of 10RM) when compared to low (33% of 10RM) and high intensities (100% of 10RM). Although the study by Jakobsen et al. (2013) was carried out with lower limbs, their findings are in line with those presented in the present study with regard to greater muscle activation for submaximal intensity loads.

When comparing changes in strength levels with training using different resistances, Calatayud et al. (2015) found similar gains for five-week training of the bench press using elastic resistance and the bench press using a Smith barbell and washers. The results of this study indicated that 6RM training for biomechanically similar movements, but performed with different resistances, generated similar strength gains. Thus, it can be inferred that by normalizing the intensity of the exercises, it is possible to obtain similar strength gains during training with elastic and fixed resistance. In addition, the ground support exercise with elastic resistance is versatile and can be performed in different locations and with different intensity settings.

According to McMaster et al. (2009), using different technologies to develop physical abilities can be a practical alternative to avoid a plateau in a training program. Anderson et al. (2008) proposed a training methodology for 44 university basketball players using fixed and variable resistance compared to a control group. Among the proposed exercises, only the squat and bench press were performed with elastic resistance in the experimental group (use of fixed and variable resistance). In the control group, all the exercises were performed with fixed resistance. The results show an interaction between the two groups, with the main effects in the maximum strength tests between the experimental and control groups. The experimental group, which used both technologies (fixed and variable resistance), obtained higher levels of strength after training for seven weeks.

However, despite the aforementioned benefits of using elastic resistance in RT, subjective load control remains one of the biggest obstacles to popularizing this type of resistance. In an attempt to normalize the load in order to make a comparison between fixed and variable resistance, the study by Melchiorri et al. (2011) performed an exhaustion protocol with dynamic and isometric elbow flexion contraction and, when comparing pre- and post-exhaustion electromyographic variables, found no significant differences. The authors justified this by the fact that the neuromuscular adaptations needed to sustain fatiguing tasks are the same for both resistances, where there is a drop in the MPF and an increase in the RMS value (Lindstrom et al., 1970, De Luca et al., 1979, Gerleman et al. 1989). In his study, Martins (2013) used a PSE validated for the use of elastic resistance (Colado et al., 2012) in order to monitor the intensity of a strength training program with elastic exercises in the elderly. Their results showed no significant difference in muscle strength variables, both in the upper and lower limbs, when compared to the control group. Despite using OMNI-RES, the author discusses the challenge and problem of quantifying the load for elastic implements.

With regard to the load control device proposed in this study, some considerations are necessary. Aggregating force signals together with electromyographic signals can be an important inferential tool in an attempt to evaluate physiological aspects of the muscular system and their consequences in terms of physical capacity development (Cannon et al., 2007; Melchiorri et al., 2011). Mechanical tests have been described in the literature as a way of quantifying different types of elastic materials. Martins et al. (2014) used a traction machine to quantify different deformations with commercial tube-shaped elastics. Simoneau et al. (2001) compared the load variation in band-shaped and tube-shaped elastics and found that despite being from the same manufacturer and material, they provided different levels of resistance for the same level of deformation. However, load quantification using traction machines does not guarantee the user objective control of intensity and applicability in the sports environment (Martins et al., 2013). Therefore, load cells, also known as force transducers, such as the one used in the device proposed in this study, can be considered an alternative for obtaining reliable control.

In this sense, the present study innovated by monitoring and controlling intensity with *biofeedback* during elastic exercise and comparing it to commercially available machinery.

No significant differences were found between the tasks performed by either group in terms of the PMFd variable. This variable is considered to be indicative of Localized Muscle Fatigue (LMF) and is justified by the increased recruitment by summation of motor units and increased power of the electromyographic signal at low frequencies when compared to high frequencies, representing a spectral signature associated with LMF (Lindstrom et al., 1970, DeLuca et al., 1979). Thus, the behavior of this variable in both groups confirms a similar pattern of fatigue for all the tasks required.

This finding corroborates Melchiorri et al. (2011) who investigated the neuromuscular changes induced by fatiguing exercise with elastic resistance compared to constant load machinery. The protocol proposed by the authors consisted of exhaustive isometric and dynamic contractions for the elbow flexion movement. Although there is no consensus on muscle fatigue in dynamic exercise compared to isometric exercise using SEMG, the authors found no significant differences in the pattern of fatigue for both contractions. Merletti and Parker (2004) and Bonato et al. (1996) associated these difficulties with the non-stationarity of the myoelectric signal. In dynamic activities, the movement artifacts of the wires and the natural movement of the skin and active muscles can influence the spectral analysis of muscle fatigue. In addition, the machinery used by the authors was made by them to perform the elbow flexion movement. Despite being a common movement among resistance training practitioners, all the results are recurrent from the execution of this exercise on a unique piece of equipment that does not exist on the market. This fact makes it difficult to apply the study by Melchiorri et al. (2011) in different training environments.

In order to add value to the analysis of the results presented by the behavior of the FPMd, the graphical method of Bland and Altman (1986) was used. This method sought to compare the agreement between the tasks regarding the fatigue pattern presented by the exercise performed on the pulley with the tasks performed with elastic resistance and objective or subjective load control. The graphs showed (figures 11 to 14) that there was excellent agreement (96.7%) between the methods (pulley vs. elastic resistance tasks) for the MPFT comparisons made. This corroborates the statistical test applied (mixed design factorial ANOVA) where the comparisons between the slopes of the regression lines infer that the fatigue presented in all the tasks for both groups was similar. This finding cancels out the speculation that the tasks performed with elastic resistance and objective or subjective load control have a greater fatiguing potential than the task performed on the pulley with a load of 30% of the CVIM during the elbow flexion exercise. In addition, as this was an exercise protocol with a limited number of twelve repetitions and submaximal intensity (30% of MVC), it was expected that the individuals taking part in the study would not be exhausted, thus justifying the similarity in the pattern of fatigue.

Considering that the tasks studied have similar indications of muscle fatigue and are different in terms of the load curve, one with fixed resistance and the other elastic, the results suggest that the adoption of exercises interspersed between these two modalities during the physical training process could become an alternative to avoid a plateau during training (Stone et al., 2000). Exercising with a single resistive method tends to promote this plateau (Fleck & Kraemer, 2006) and minimize the desired results (Stone et al., 2000).

As for the level of muscle activation, the non-significance between the tasks in the GBIO group suggests that by having objective load control in variable resistances, the intensity of the exercise remains sufficiently equivalent to the task that uses fixed resistance, enabling similar gains in muscle strength and/or endurance (Calatayud et al., 2015). The absence of quantitative load control for elastic implements prevents the evolutionary monitoring of RT, in addition to prescribing the load required to achieve the proposed goal (Tan, 1999; Fleck & Kraemer, 2006; McMaster et al., 2009). The objective load control device for elastic resistance used in the present study encourages the use of elastic implements by achieving similar levels of muscle activation when exercising with a fixed load. In practical terms, the use of the device reinforces the portability of the elastic as well as becoming a low-cost training variation alternative compared to machinery (Anderson et al., 2008; Melchiorri et al., 2011; Martins et al., 2014).

CHAPTER 6 - CONCLUSIONS

Subjective load control for exercises with an elastic implement did not guarantee that the level of muscle activation (RMS) was the same as for tasks with fixed resistance. Furthermore, when using this type of control, even in individuals familiar with resistance training, the load of the elbow flexion exercise with an elastic implement was underestimated.

The level of muscle activation with objective load control for elastic resistance with *biofeedback* was similar to the task with fixed resistance. This control allowed better monitoring of the intensity (load) and maintenance of the movement pattern in the elbow flexion exercise.

Furthermore, the behavior of the FPMd was similar for both groups in all tasks and showed a similar level of fatigue.

The positive results found with the use of a load control device with *biofeedback* confirm the use of elastic resistance in the development of different physical capacities and make it possible to use a variety of implements in physical training associated with portability, low cost and better control of movement technique. Further studies involving strength curves, methodological proposals for comparing different types of resistance and the chronic effects of using elastic implements with load control and *biofeedback* are also suggested.

BIBLIOGRAPHICAL REFERENCES

ACSM - American College of Sports Medicine (2009). Position Statement: **Exercise and physical activity for older adults. Medicine and Science in Sports and Exercise**, 41 (7): 1510-1530.

AAGAARD P, SIMONSEN EB, ANDERSEN JL, MAGNUSSON P, DYHRE-POULSEN P. (2002). Increased rate of force development and neural drive of human skeletal muscle following resistance training. **J Appl Physiol,** 93(4):1318-26.

ALKNER BA, TESCH PA, BERG HE. (2000). Quadriceps EMG/force relationship in knee extension and leg press. **Med Sci Sports Exerc**, 32(2), 459-463.

ANDERS, C., BRETSCHNEIDER, S., BERNSDORF, A., & SCHNEIDER, W. (2005). Activation characteristics of shoulder muscles during maximal and submaximal efforts. **Eur J Appl Physiol**, 93(5-6), 540-546.

ANDERSEN LL, ANDERSEN CH, MORTENSEN OS, POULSEN OM, BJOMLUND IBT, ZEBIS MK. (2010). Muscle activation and perceived loading during rehabilitation exercises: comparison of dumbbells and elastic resistance. **Physical Therapy**, 90:538-549.

ANDERSON, CE; SFORZO GA; SIGG, JA. (2008). The Effects of Combining Elastic and Free Weight Resistance on Strength and Power in Athletes. **Journal of Strength and Conditioning Research**, 22(2):567-574

ANDRADE MM, TELES FS, ROCHA VA, MARTINS WR, OLIVEIRA, RJ, Inventores; (2014) Fundaçâo Universidade de Brasilia (FUB); assignee.

***Biofeedback* System for the Practice of Resistance Exercises with Elastic Overload**. Brazil, BR Patent 1020140072322.

ANDRADE MM. (2006). **Time-frequency analysis of electromyographic signals to assess muscle fatigue on a cycle ergometer**. Doctoral thesis, ENE/UnB.

AZEVEDO, FM. (2003). **Study of the force and electrical activity generated by the quadriceps femoris muscle submitted to elastic resistance exercises**. Master's dissertation, Bioengineering/USP Sâo Carlos.

BILODEAU M, SCHINDLER-IVENS S, WILLIAMS DM, CHANDRAN R, SHARMA SS. (2003). EMG frequency contente changes with increasing force during fatigue in the quadriceps femoris muscle of men and women. **J Electromyogr Kinesiol**, 13(1), 83-92

BLAND, JM; ALTMAN, DG. (1986). Statistical methods for assessing agreement between two methods of clinical measurement. **Lancet**, i:307-310

BONATO P, GAGLIATI G, KNAFLITZ M. (1996) Analysis of myoelectric signals recorded during dynamic contractions. **Engineering in Medicine and Biology Magazine,** IEEE, 15(6), 102-11.

BOTTARO M RA, OLIVEIRA RJ. (2005). The effects of rest interval on quadriceps torque during an isokinetic testing protocol in elderly. **Journal of Sports Science and Medicine**, 4:285-90.

CALATAYUD J, BORREANI S, COLADO JC, MARTIN F, TELLA V, ANDERSEN LL. (2015). Bench press and push-up at comparable levels of muscle activity results in similar strength gains. **Journal of Strength and Conditioning Research**, 29(1):246-253.

CANNON J, KAY D, TARPENNING KM, MARINO FE. (2007). Comparative effects of resistance training on peak isometric torque, muscle hypertrophy, voluntary activation and surface EMG between young and elderly women. **Clin Physiol Funct Imaging**, 27:91-100.

CARMO JC. (2003). **Development of dedicated instrumentation and proposal of a technique for analyzing fatigue in cyclists using wavelet transforms**. PhD thesis, ENE/UnB.

CLANCY EA, MORIN EL, MERLETTI, R. (2002). Sampling, noise-reduction and amplitude estimation issues in surface electromyography. **J Electromyogr**

Kinesiol, 12(1); 1-16.

COLADO JC, TRIPLETT NT. (2008). Effects of a short-term resistance program using elastic bands versus weight machines for sedentary middleaged women. **Journal of strength and conditioning research**, 22(5):1441- 8

COLADO JC, TRIPLETT NT, TELLA V, SAUCEDO P, ABELLAN J. (2009). Effects of aquatic resistance training on health and fitness in postmenopausal women. **European Journal of Applied Physiology**, 106: 113-122.

COLADO JC, GARCIA-MASSO X, PELLICER M, ALAKHDAR Y, BENAVENT J, CABEZA- RUIZ R. (2011). A comparison of elastic tubing and isotonic resistance exercises. **International Journal of Sports and Medicine**, 31: 810-817.

COLADO JC, GARCIA-MASSO X, TRIPLETT TN, FLANDEZ J, BORREANI S, TELLA V. (2012). Concurrent validation of the OMNI-resistance exercise scale of perceived exertion with Thera-band resistance bands. **Journal of Strength and Conditioning Research**, 26(11): 3018-24.

CHAFFIN, DB. (1973) Localized Muscle Fatigue - Definition and Measurement. **Journal of Occupational Medicine**, 15(4): 346-354.

CHRISTENSEN H, SOGAARD K, JENSEN BR. (1995) Intramuscular and surface EMG power spectrum from dynamic and static contractions. **J Electr Kinesiol,** 5(1), 27-36.

DE LUCA, CJ. Physiology and Mathematics of Myoelectric Signal. (1979) **IEEE Transactions on Biomedical Engineering**, 26(6), 313-325.

DE LUCA, CJ. The use of surface electromyography in biomechanics. (1997) **J Applied Biomechanics**. 13, 135-163

DE LUCA, CJ. (2002). Surface electromyography detection and recording. ***DelSys Incorporated***.

DE LUCA, CJ. (2003). Fundamental Concepts in EMG Signal Acquisition.

***DelSys Incorporated*.**

DE LUCA, CJ. (2006). Electromyography. **Encyclopedia of Medical Devices and Instrumentation**, 98-109.

ERFANIAN A, CHIZECK HJ, HASHEMI RM. (1994). Evoked EMG in electrically stimulated muscle and mechanisms of fatigue. **Engineering in Medicine and Biology Society**, in 16th Annual International Conference of the IEEE.

FARINA D, MERLETTI R, RAINOLDI A, BUINOCORE M. (1999). Two methods for the measurement of voluntary contraction torque in biceps brachii muscle. **Medical Engineering & Physics**, 21, 533-540.

FARINA D, GAZZONI M, CAMELIA F (2004). Methods for estimating muscle fiber conduction velocity from surface electromyographic signals. **Med Biol Eng Comput**, 42(4), 432-445.

FARINA D, POZZO M, MERLO E, BOTTIN A, MERLETTI R (2004c). Assessment of average muscle fiber conduction velocity from surface EMG signals during fatiguing dynamic contractions. **IEEE Trans Biomed Eng**, 51(8), 1383-1393.

FIELD, A. **Discovering statistics using SPSS**. (2009). Translation by Lori Viali, 2 editions, Porto Alegre: Artmed, 688p.

FLECK SJ, KRAEMER WJ. (2004). **Designing Resistance Programs**. 3 edition, Champaign, IL: Human Kinectics, p.31.

FLECK SJ, KRAEMER WJ. (2006). **Fundamentals of Muscle Strength Training**. Translated by Jerri Luiz Ribeiro, 3 editions, Porto Alegre: Artmed, 376p.

FULLER GD. ***Biofeedback*: Methods and procedures in clinical practice** (1977). San Francisco: *Biofeedback* Press, 343p.

GERLEMAN, D. G., AND COOK, T. M. (1989) Instrumentation, in manual of surface electromyography for use in the occupational setting, **DHHS Publication**, US, pp. 81-126.

HALL, SJ. **Basic Biomechanics** (2000) 3ed. Rio de Janeiro, Guanabara Koogan, 415p.

HERMENS HJ, FRERIKS B, DISSELHORST-KLUG C, AND RAU G. (2000). Development of recommendations for SEMG sensors and sensor placement procedures. **J Electromyogr Kinesiol**, 10: 361-374.

HUNTER, GR; WETZSTEIN, CJ; MCLAFFERTY, CL; ZUCKERMAN, PA; LANDERS, KA; BAMMAN, MM. (2001). High-resistance versus variable-resistance training in older adults. **Medicine & Science in Sports Exercise**; 33(10)1759-1764

JAKOBSEN, MD, SUNDSTRUP E, ANDERSEN CH, PERSSON R, ZEBIS MK, ANDERSEN LL. (2014). Effectiveness of hamstring knee rehabilitation exercise performed in training machine vc. Elastic resistance. **Am J Phys Med Rehabil**, 93(4).

KRAEMER WJ, ADAMS K, CAFARELLI E, DUDLEY GA, DOOLY C, FEIGENBAUM M. (2002). American College of Sports Medicine position stand. Progression models in resistance training for health adults. **Med Sci Sports Exerc**, 34(1), 364-380.

KONRAD, P. (2005). The ABC of EMG - A Practical Introduction to Kinesiological Electromyography. ***Noraxon Inc.*** *USA*, 1-60.

LEEDHAM JS, DOWLING JJ. (1995). Force-length, torque-angle and EMG-joint angle relationships of the human in vivo biceps brachii. **Eur J Appli. Physiol**, (70): 421-426.

LINDSTROM, L.; PETERSEN, I. (1970). Power spectrum analysis of EMG signals and its application. In Desmedt JE (Ed): **Computer-Aided Electromyography: Progress in Clinical Neurophysiology**. Basel, Switzerland, Karger, v.10, p.5.

MANNING, RJ; GRAVES, JE, CARPENTER DM; LEGGETT SH; POLLOCK ML. (1989). Constant vs Variable resistance knee extension training. **Medicine and Science in Sports and Exercise**, 22(3), 397-401.

MARTINS WR OR, CARVALHO RS, DAMASCENO V, SANTOS M. (2013). Elastic resistance training to Increase Muscle Strength in Elderly: A systematic review with meta-analysis. **Archives of Gerontology and Geriatrics**, 57(1): 8-15.

MARTINS WR. (2013) **Effects of Short-term Elastic Resistance Training on Strength and Muscle Mass in Demented Elderly**. Doctoral Thesis.

MARTINS WR, CARVALHO RS, SILVA MS, BLASCZYK JC, ARAÙJO JA, CARMO JC, RODACKI ALF, OLIVEIRA RJ. (2014). Mechanical evaluation of elastic tubes used in physical therapy. **Physiother Theory Pract**, 30(3): 21822.

MASUDA T, KIZUKA T, ZHE JY, YAMADA H, SAITOU K, SADOYAMA T. (2001). Influence of contraction force and speed on mucle fiber conduction velocity during dynamic voluntary exercise. **J Electromyogr Kinesiol**, 11(2), 85-94

MARCHETTI PH, DUARTE M. (2006) **Instrumentaçâo em Eletromiografia**. Biophysics Laboratory. Handout.

MCARDLE, WD, KATCH, FI, KATCH, VL. (2008). **Exercise physiology: energy, nutrition and human performance**. 6ª edition, Rio de Janeiro: Ed. Guanabara Koogan.

MCMASTER, DT; CRONIN J, MCGUIGAN M. (2009) Forms of Variable Resistance Training. **Strength and Conditioning Journal**, 31(1): 50-64.

MELCHIORRI, G; RAINOLDI, A. (2011). Muscle fatigue induced by two different resistances: Elastic tubing versus weight machines. **Journal of Electromyography and Kinesiology**, 21(6): 954-959.

MERLETTI, R., DI TORINO, P. (1999). Standards for reporting EMG data. **J**

Elec. Kines, 9(1): III-IV.

MERLETTI, R., PARKER, P. (2004). Electromyography: physiology, engineering, and noninvasive applications [Hoboken, NJ]: **IEEE/ John Wiley & Sons**.

MEZZARANE RA, ELIAS LA, MAGALHÀES FH, CHAUD VM AND KOHN AF. (2014). **Experimental and simulated EMG responses in the study of the human spinal cord**. Electrodiagnosis in New Frontiers of Clinical Research. São Paulo, Chapter 4, 57-87.

MORAS G, RODRÎGUEZ-JIMÉNEZ S, BUSQUETS A, TOUS-FAJARDO J, POZZO M, MUJIKA I. (2009). A metronome for controlling the mean velocity during the bench press exercise. **Journal of strength and conditioning research**, 23(3), 926-931.

MORITANI T, MURO M. (1987). Motor unit activity and surface electromyogram power spectrum during increasing force of contraction. **Eur J Appl Physiol Occup Physiol**, 56(3), 260-265.

MYLES, PS; CUI, J. (2007). Using the Bland-Altman method to measure agreement with repeated measures. **British Journal of Anaesthesia**, 99(3): 309-11.

OLIVEIRA AS, GONÇALVES M. (2009). Posiotioning during resistance elbow flexor exercise affects electromyographic activity, heart rate, and perceived exertion. **Journal of Strength and Conditioning Research**, 23(3), 854-862.

PEREIRA, MC. (2009). **Relationship of electromyographic parameters with aerobic-anaerobic transition in trained cyclists.** Master's dissertation.

PETERSON MD, RHEA MR, SEN A, GORDON PM. (2010). Resistance exercise for muscular strength in older adults: a meta-analysis. **Ageing Res Rev**, 9(3):226-37.

PRESTES J, DE LIMA C, FROLLINI AB, DONATTO FF, CONTE M. (2009). Comparison of linear and reverse linear periodization effects on maximal strength and body composition. **Journal of Strength and Conditioning Research**, 23(1), 266-274

ROBERTSON RJ, GOSS FL, RUTKOWSKI J, LENZ B, DIXON C, TIMMER J. (2003). Concurrent validation of the OMNI perceived exertion scale for resistance exercise. **Medicine and science in sports and exercise**, 35(2):333-41.

ROCHA JÛNIOR, VA. (2008) **Neuromuscular responses of the vastus lateralis muscle to the adapted pre-exhaustion method**. Master's dissertation.

ROSA DE SA AA, SOARES AB. 3D computer interface for real-time multimodal *biofeedback* (2012). **Brazilian Journal of Biomedical Engineering**, 28(4), 387-397.

SAKANOUE N, KATAYAMA K. (2007). The resistance quantity in knee extension movement of exercise bands (Thera-Band). **Journal of Physical Therapy Science**, 19: 287-291.

SCHOENFELD, BJ. (2010). Mechanisms of muscle hypertrophy and their application to resistance training. **Journal of Strength and Conditioning Research,** 24(10), 2857-2872.

SCHWANBECK S, CHILIBECK PD, BINSTED G. (2009). A comparison of free weight squat to smith machine squat using electromyography. **Journal of Strength and Conditioning Research**, 23(9), 2588-2591.

SIMONEAU GG, BEREDA SM, SOBUSH DC, STARSKY AJ. (2001). Biomechanics of elastic resistance in therapeutic exercise programs. **The Journal of orthopaedic and sports physical therapy**, 31(1):16-24.

SOARES, FA. (2013). **Surface electromyographic signal processing using image processing techniques**. Doctoral thesis.

STEIB, S; SCHOENE, D; PFEIFER, K. Dose-response relationship of resistance training in older adults: a meta-analysis. (2010) **Med Sci Sports**

Exerc, 42(5):902-14.

SUNDSTRUP E, JAKOBSEN MD, ANDERSEN CH, ZEBIS MK, MORTENSEN OS, ANDERSEN LL. (2012). **Journal of strength and conditioning research**, 26(7), p. 1897-1903.

TAN, B. (1999). Manipulating resistance training program variables to optimize maximum strength in men: a review. **Journal of Strength and Conditioning Research**,13(3), 289-304.

WEBSTER JG. (1984). Reducing motion artifacts and interference in biopotential recording. **IEEE Trans Biomed Eng**, 31(12), 823-826.

WELSCH EA, BIRD M, MAYHEW JL. (2005). Electromyography activity of the pectoralis major and anterior deltoid muscles during three upper-body lifts. **Journal of Strength and Conditioning Research**, 19(2), 449-452.

ANNEX

ANNEX I

TERM OF FREE AND INFORMED CONSENT (TCLE)

Dear participant, you are being invited to voluntarily take part in a research project at the University of Brasilia entitled "Methodological Proposals Applied to Physical Exercises with Elastic Resistance".

Nowadays, the use of elastic bands for physical exercise is growing, often very similar to traditional weight training. However, unlike with weights, control of the load of elastic exercises is either non-existent or done through the perception of the student and/or teacher. Thus, the lack of load control does not always guarantee gains in training or even whether the exercise is being performed at the proposed intensity. With this in mind, the aim of this research is to propose a methodology for exercises performed with elastic bands using a device to adjust the load during the execution of the exercises and to compare muscle parameters between elastic resistance and the pulley.

It is hoped that exercises with load control on elastic bands will be able to accentuate the benefits of the exercise, as well as providing control of execution and guaranteeing intensity, as occurs in exercises with weight machines.

Please read the information contained in this form carefully before making any decisions about your participation as a volunteer. Any clarifications you feel are necessary before and during the research can be made directly to the researcher in charge. In the same way, you have the right to refuse to answer questions that embarrass you. Your participation is voluntary and you will have complete and total freedom to withdraw from the study at any time, without any harm to you. All information related to the research is confidential and any information disclosed in a report or publication will be done so in coded form, so that your confidentiality is maintained. The researchers guarantee that your name will not be disclosed under any circumstances in any publication.

The research involves two (2) tests: (1) evaluation of the maximum voluntary isometric contraction of the elbow flexion movement and (2) execution of a protocol of 12 repetitions of the elbow flexion movement with two types of resistance: pulley and elastic. This stage will last one day, meaning that you will only need to come to the collection laboratory for one day.

All the research will be carried out at the University of Brasilia, located on the Darcy Ribeiro University Campus, Brasilia, DF - CEP 70910-900, and specifically at the Biological Signal Processing and Motor Control Laboratory of the Faculty of Physical Education. This consent form is written in two copies, one for the participant and one for the researcher, and must be signed by both parties. If you have any questions, you can contact the researcher in charge, Prof. Fernanda Teles, by telephone: 619961-4907; or by e-mail: fernandasteles@hotmail.com. You can also contact the Research Ethics Committee of the Faculty of Health Sciences of the University of Brasilia directly by telephone: (61) 31071947; or by e-mail: cepfs@unb.br.

Name / signature

Researcher in Charge

Brasilia,from

ANNEX II - Electrogoniometer Calibration Algorithm

```
clear all

close all

clc

cd '/Users/sidneiteles/Fernanda/Faculdade_UnB/MESTRADO/dados mestrado/Coleta New 26-02-15';

fs = 2000;

v_color = ['bkrgymcbkrgymcbkrgymcbkrgymcbkrgymc'];
```

```
% INCLUDE INTEGERS FOR DIVISION

clc

sit = {['gtrdm'] ['gtrdi'] ['polia']}; %Set up experimental situations

for i = 1 : length(sit);

c_load = ['load suj19_',sit{i},'.txt']; %Loads signals

eval(c_load);

end for i = 1 : length(sit);

c_filt1 = ['suj19_',sit{i},'_filt(:,1 : 2) = butter_low(suj19_',sit{i},'(:, 1:2), fs);'];
%Filters force and goniometer signals

eval(c_filt1);

c_filt2 = ['suj19_',sit{i},'_filt(:, 3: 4 ) =

butter4_20_500(detrend(suj19_',sit{i},'(:, 3:4),"constant"), fs);']; %Filters emg
signals

eval(c_filt2);

end

goni1 = [20 30:20:170 180]; %Set goniometer vectors

for i = 1 : length(goni1);

goni2{i} = num2str(goni1(i));

end for i = 1 : length(goni2);

c_load = ['load calgoni',goni2{i},'.txt']; %Load signals eval(c_load);

c_goni = ['vector_goni(i) = mean(calgoni',goni2{i},');'];

eval(c_goni);

end

%Upload goni data

vector_goni_cal = [20 30 50 70 90 110 130 150 170 180];
```

```
load_goni = {['20']; ['30']; ['50']; ['70']; ['90']; ['110']; ['130']; ['150']; ['170'];
['180']};
for i = 1 : length(load_goni);
command_load = ['cal_goni{i}= load(''calgoni',load_goni{i},'.txt'');'];
eval(command_load);
command_cut = ['calgoni',load_goni{i},' =
calgoni',load_goni{i},'(500:1000);'];
eval(command_cut);
command_filt = ['tension_goni(i) = mean(butter_low(calgoni',load_goni{i},',
fs));'];
eval(command_filt)
end
%Calibration goni
p = polyfit(tension_goni, vector_goni_cal, 1);
calibrated_straight = polyval(p, tension_goni);
straight = (vector_goni_cal - p(2))/p(1);
straight_plot = polyval(p, straight);
plot(calibrated_straight,'r*-');
hold on;
plot(straight_plot,'*-');
pause;
close;
```

ANNEX III - Algorithm for Cutting Signals by the Electrogoniometer

```
%Cut the signals;
```

```
bulhas_gtrdi_angulo = fases_goni_fe_angulo(goni_cal_gtrdi, suj19_gtrdi_filt(:,3));
title('GtrdI CROWNED BY ANGLE');
figure;
bulhas_gtrdm_angulo = fases_goni_fe_angulo(goni_cal_gtrdm, suj19_gtrdm_filt(:,3));
title('GtrdM CROWNED BY ANGLE');
figure;
bulhas_polia_angulo = fases_goni_fe_angulo(goni_cal_polia, suj19_polia_filt(:,3));
title('POLY CUT BY ANGLE');
```

ANNEX IV - Algorithm for Calculating Electromyographic Variables (RMS and FPMd)

```
for i = 1 : length(bulhas_gtrdi_angulo)
rms_gtrdi_angulo(i) = rms2(bulhas_gtrdi_angulo{i});
mdf_gtrdi_angulo(i) = freq_median(bulhas_gtrdi_angulo{i}, fs);
aux=bulhas_gtrdi_angulo{i};
end
gtrdim = mean (gtrdi);
clear aux
for i = 1 : length(bulhas_gtrdm_angulo)
rms_gtrdm_angulo(i) = rms2(bulhas_gtrdm_angulo{i});
mdf_gtrdm_angulo(i) = freq_median(bulhas_gtrdm_angulo{i}, fs);
aux=bulhas_gtrdm_angulo{i};
end
```

```
gtrdmm = mean (gtrdi);
clear aux
for i = 1 : length(bulhas_polia_angulo)
rms_polia_angulo(i) = rms2(bulhas_polia_angulo{i});
mdf_polia_angulo(i) = freq_median(bulhas_polia_angulo{i}, fs);
aux=bulhas_polia_angulo{i};
end
poliam = mean (pulley);
clc
rms_gtrdi_angulo = rms_gtrdi_angulo'
mdf_gtrdi_angulo = mdf_gtrdi_angulo'
rms_gtrdm_angulo = rms_gtrdm_angulo'
mdf_gtrdm_angulo = mdf_gtrdm_angulo'
rms_polia_angulo = rms_polia_angulo'
mdf_polia_angulo = mdf_polia_angulo'
```

ANNEX V - Algorithm for Calculating the Frequency Spectrum of the Electromyographic Signal

```
pause;
close all;
for i = 1 : length(sit);
command_freq = ['freq(suj19_',sit{i},'_filt(:, 3), fs, v_color(i));']; %Filters signals
force and goniometer
eval(command_freq);
command_title = ['title(''Signal frequency response - Situation ',sit{i},''');'];
```

```
eval(command_title);

pause;

close;

end
```

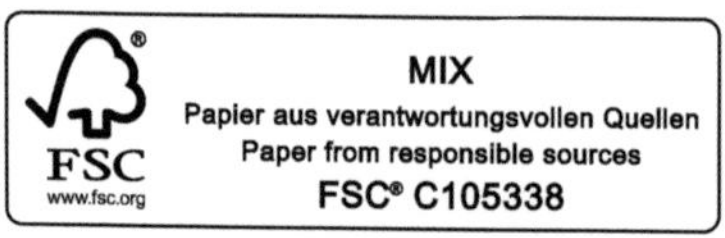

Printed by Books on Demand GmbH, Norderstedt / Germany